# YOUR KNOWLEDGE HAS VALUE

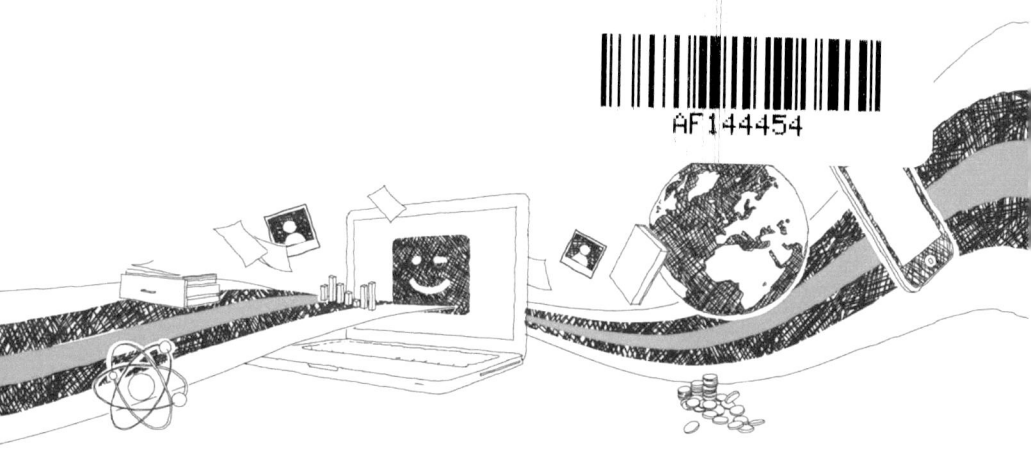

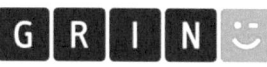

**Bibliographic information published by the German National Library:**

The German National Library lists this publication in the National Bibliography; detailed bibliographic data are available on the Internet at http://dnb.dnb.de .

**Imprint:**

Copyright © 2012 GRIN Verlag, Open Publishing GmbH
Print and binding: Books on Demand GmbH, Norderstedt Germany
ISBN: 978-3-668-02110-5

**This book at GRIN:**

http://www.grin.com/en/e-book/303800/impact-of-advances-in-medical-technology-on-health-care-costs

Ed Malo

# Impact of Advances in Medical Technology on Health Care Costs

GRIN Publishing

**GRIN - Your knowledge has value**

Since its foundation in 1998, GRIN has specialized in publishing academic texts by students, college teachers and other academics as e-book and printed book. The website www.grin.com is an ideal platform for presenting term papers, final papers, scientific essays, dissertations and specialist books.

**Visit us on the internet:**

http://www.grin.com/

http://www.facebook.com/grincom

http://www.twitter.com/grin_com

# The Impact of Advances in Medical Technology on Health Care Costs

*Edward Malo, B.S.B.A*

**Cameron University**

**MBA Candidate**

**Lawton, OK**

**Abstract**

*The purpose of this paper is to examine the impact of advances in medical technology on health care costs in the United States. More specifically, this paper provides an overview of just some of the plethora of compelling evidence in the public forum, presented by experts in fields related to this topic which do in fact appear to show the correlation exists. An overview of the changes in health care related expenses and some of the advances in medical technology is also provided for background.*

# Table of Contents

## Introduction

Health care costs in the United States continue to rise at alarming rates. As many citizens, politicians, physicians, government policy makers and others speculate as to the causes, some have theorized and studied the impact advances in medical technology have had on the rising costs. Findings are mixed across different articles but case studies by two experts provide some compelling evidence on this theory. One case study shows how medical technology can be part of a sometimes extended and wasteful treatment plan for patients, while the other shows how advanced medical technology can actually reduce treatment costs by preventing unnecessary and costly procedures.

Another facet to explore in any topic such as rising health care costs, where it is so widely discussed and debated by average people, is the public perception of medical technology and its role in this. This is also presented in this paper with a brief overview of a survey conducted by Harvard University in conjunction with other organizations.

First, facts about rising health care costs are briefly presented along with an overview of some of the major advances in medical technology to provide background information. A majority of the paper is devoted to the literature selected for relevance and case studies taken from presentations by experts in related fields. Selected literature is reviewed with summaries of the authors' relevant contributions to the topic highlighted and the chosen case studies are described in detail. Lastly, there is a brief discussion of some of the observed findings in the literature reviewed and opinions for directions for future explorations of this topic are given.

## Background

According to the National Coalition on Health Care (2007), the United States as a nation spent $2 Trillion in 2005 on health care alone, which represented a 6.9% increase over the previous year. That rate is two times the rate of inflation and that amount is 16% of the nation's Gross Domestic Product (GDP). Comparatively, health care accounts for 9.7% of GDP in Canada, 9.5% in France and 10.7% in Germany.

Health insurance premiums for both employers and employees are also on the rise. In 2006, larger employers saw an increase of 7.7% in their health insurance premiums, smaller firms averaged 8.8%, and the smallest (less than 24 employees) had their premiums increase by 10.5%. Finally, while wages between 2000 and 2006 increased by approximately 20%, employment-based health insurance premiums increased by 87% during the same time period. American workers, on average paid $1,094 per year more for family coverage in 2006 than they did in 2000. Also since 2000, the average employee contribution to their employer's health insurance program has increased by over 143% between 2000 and 2006 (National Coalition on Health Care, 2007).

**Figure 1**

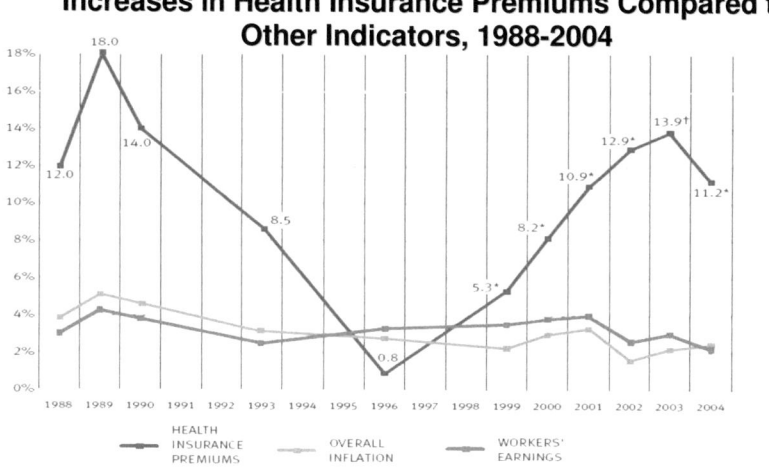

Source: Controlling Health care Costs (Gilbertson, 2005).

Figure 1 (above) shows the changes in health insurance premiums between 1988 and 2004 compared to other indicators such as overall inflation and workers' earnings (Gilbertson, 2005).

Over the past two-hundred and fifty years mankind has made enormous advances in medical technology. From the advent of vaccinations and antibiotics, to the discovery of x-ray

5

technology and the perfecting of heart transplant surgery, the discoveries and advancements vary widely. A brief overview of some of those major advances is presented in Figure 2.

**Figure 2**

```
┌─────────────────────────────────────────────────────────────────────────────────┐
│ Advances in Medical Technology over the Last 250 Years                            │
│                                                                                   │
│ 1796 – Vaccines are used for the first time.                                      │
│ 1865 – Antiseptics are used for the first time in surgery.                        │
│ 1895 – The world's first X-Ray is taken.                                          │
│ 1897 – Aspirin is invented.                                                       │
│ 1905 – The research that led to administering Vitamins started.                   │
│ 1922 – Insulin to treat diabetes patients is discovered.                          │
│ 1928 – Penicillin is discovered.                                                  │
│ 1933 – Research starts that leads to the development of CPR.                      │
│ 1936 – Nuclear Medicine is born when Radiation is used to treat disease for the first time. │
│ 1946 – Following WWII, the first Chemotherapy drugs are discovered.               │
│ 1953 – The vaccination for Polio is discovered.                                   │
│ 1957 – The brain EEG Toposcope is invented.                                       │
│ 1958 – The Ultrasound is first used on a pregnant woman.                          │
│ 1960 – The world's first totally internal pacemaker was created.                  │
│ 1965 – The first Portable Defibrillator is installed.                             │
│ 1967 – The first human Heart Transplant is performed.                             │
│ 1972 – The CAT scan was first introduced.                                         │
│ 1980 – Smallpox is officially eradicated from the world.                          │
│ 1981 – The MRI was first introduced.                                              │
│ 1982 – The world's first permanent Artificial Heart is implanted into a human.    │
│ 1987 – The first Laser Eye Surgery was performed on a patient.                    │
│ 1990 – Scientists begin mapping the Human Genome.                                 │
│ 1997 – Dolly the sheep becomes the first Cloned animal.                           │
│ 1998 – A biologist produces the first line of viable human Stem Cells.            │
│ 2000 – The PET Scan is introduced.                                                │
│ 2003 – Scientist complete mapping of the entire Human Genome.                     │
└─────────────────────────────────────────────────────────────────────────────────┘
```

Sources: Timeline of Medical Breakthroughs (Olund, 2008), Dec. 24, 1936: Radiation Used to Treat Disease for the First Time (Long, 2007), Who discovered chemotheraphy (Cancer Research UK Charity, 2007) and Stages of Medicine (Regio, n.d.)

Some of these technological advances shown in Figure 2 are identified in the literature reviewed and case studies discussed later in this paper.

## Literature Review

Annamarie Barros, M.A. (1995) among many things, is a laboratory operations adviser for Ernst & Young's north central region of the United States. In an article Barros wrote for the Medical Laboratory Observer she discusses laboratories across the US that she has observed stuck in wastefull practices with no regard for costs. That disregard translates into higher prices charged patients and hospitals for laboratory work. However Barros identified obsolete equipment in laboatories as one of the most common ways for waste to occur. Believing older equipment is more reliable, still functioning sufficiently and less costly then replacing it with newer technology, these laboratories waste time for patient care and money in terms of the direct and indirect costs they fail to notice associated with the outdated equipment. She also identified other sources of waste. For example, the misuse of skills when laboratories under utilize technicians and have actual scientists performing technician functions and a lack of focus on an "effective patient outcome" which she describes as laboratories doing things correct the first time, and insisting on only relevant laboratory work with the best interests of the actual patient in mind for turn around time, costs and more (Barros, 1995).

News-Medical.net (2007), an online medical news service published an article about a paper writen by Rita Redberg, M.D. from the University of California, San Francisco's Medical Center. The paper addressed the role advances in medical technology were playing on rising health care costs and the lack of an "evidence-based system" to evaluate new medical technologies and their net benefit in terms of costs to the patients. The article highlights Dr. Redberg's example of Computed Tomography Angiography (CTA) as an example of new and expensive technology experiencing widespread acceptance and use due to increased phycision and patient demand coupled with media attention "despite little evidence showing CTA leads to better patient care than alternative procedures" (News-Medical.net, 2007).

Steve Lohr (2004) of the New York Times wrote an article about medical technology's unique role in increasing health care costs. That unique role, as described by Lohr is that advances in medical technology have caused people's life spans to increase and people who live longer require more health care than those who die at young ages. Improvements in medical technology are also in high demand, and have been for many years by physicians and patients alike. There is an overwhelming desire to have technology that can provide benefits such as finding illnesses sooner and treating patients faster and less obtrusively. So in short, according to Lohr and what he found by speaking with health care economists, physicians turned entrepreneurs and medical technology analysts just to name a few, is that expensive medical technology in the form of drugs, surgical implants, detection equipment and more in constant high demand will continue to improve our standards of living and lengthen our lives, with higher health care costs as a necessary side effect (Lohr, 2004).

ScienceDaily wrote a review of an article published by The University of Michigan (1998) titled *Managed Care, Medical Technology, and Health Care Cost Growth: A Review of the Evidence* in which they examined evidence to find the relationship between both "managed care" practices and medical technology on rising health care costs. One of the authors of the article, Michael E. Chernew, a public health economist summarized the University's findings with regards to medical technology's role in a quote to ScienceDaily, "The reason why health care costs are higher now than they have been in the past is because of new medical technology. It's not increased waste, it's not fraud, it's not increased law suits, it's not the fact that people on average are older---all of that may contribute, but the predominant factor relates to the development and utilization of new medical techniques, of which there are an enormous number" (University Of Michigan, 1998).

Thomas Bodenheimer, M.D. (2005) wrote an article titled *High and Rising Health Care Costs. Part 2: Technologic Innovation* in the Medical and Public Issues Journal, Volume 142, Number 11 edition. In the article, Bodenheimer discusses the main driving forces behind medical technology's contribution to rising health care costs. He cites the increased availability and heavy promotion of new medical technologies, physicians more ready to accept new technology for various reasons including a lack of knowledge as to the actual benefits and the higher fees charged for use of the latest technology in diagnosis, a lack of regulatory constraints in terms of costs and efficiency and increasing public demand and thirst for new and better technology and use of that technology as some of the factors creating, medical technology's sizeable impact on rising health care costs (Bodenheimer, 2005).

Public perspective of the impact advances in medical technology are having on rising health care costs is important and worthy of exploration. In August of 2005, Harvard University in conjunction with USA Today and the Kaiser Family Foundation conducted a survey and analyzed the results to examine health care issues. The survey, among many things tested

8

people's perceptions as to the reasons why health care costs are rising. The results of that question are displayed in Figure 3:

**Figure 3**

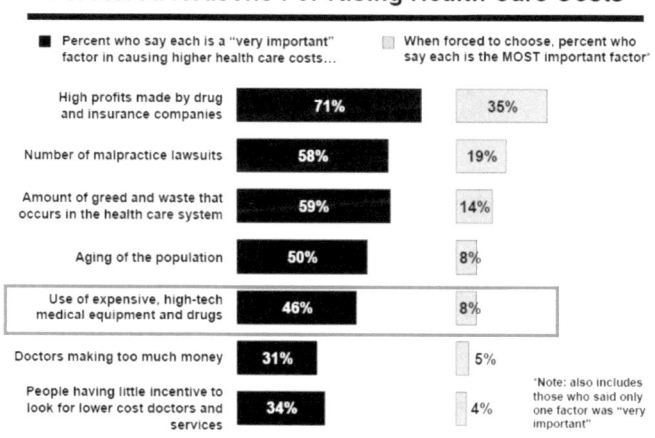

## Perceived Reasons For Rising Health Care Costs

| | Percent who say each is a "very important" factor in causing higher health care costs... | When forced to choose, percent who say each is the MOST important factor* |
|---|---|---|
| High profits made by drug and insurance companies | 71% | 35% |
| Number of malpractice lawsuits | 58% | 19% |
| Amount of greed and waste that occurs in the health care system | 59% | 14% |
| Aging of the population | 50% | 8% |
| Use of expensive, high-tech medical equipment and drugs | 46% | 8% |
| Doctors making too much money | 31% | 5% |
| People having little incentive to look for lower cost doctors and services | 34% | 4% |

*Note: also includes those who said only one factor was "very important"

Source: Health care Costs Survey (Harvard University Project, 2005)

Of those surveyed, 46% say that the use of expensive, high-tech medical equipment and drugs is a "very important" factor in causing higher health care costs. When respondents were forced to choose the most important factor causing higher health care costs, the use of expensive, high-tech medical equipment and drugs was chosen by only 8% of them though. A majority of those who took the survey, 35% choose high profits made by drug and insurance companies as the most important factor (Harvard University, 2005).

## Case Studies

In her presentation to the Citizens' Health Care Working Group in July of 2005, Elizabeth B. Gilbertson, the Director of Strategic Planning and Public Policy for the Hotel Employees and Restaurant Employees International Union Welfare Fund described the cost of health care as 85% composed of what doctors do themselves or order to be done to treat a patient. She then presented the result of her case study where three different doctors were hypothetically presented

9

with a sick patient with a set of symptoms and each presented a different treatment plan based on their own experience, personal treatment styles, knowledge and usage habits of medical technology, etc. Figure 4 summarizes the case study and its results.

**Figure 4**

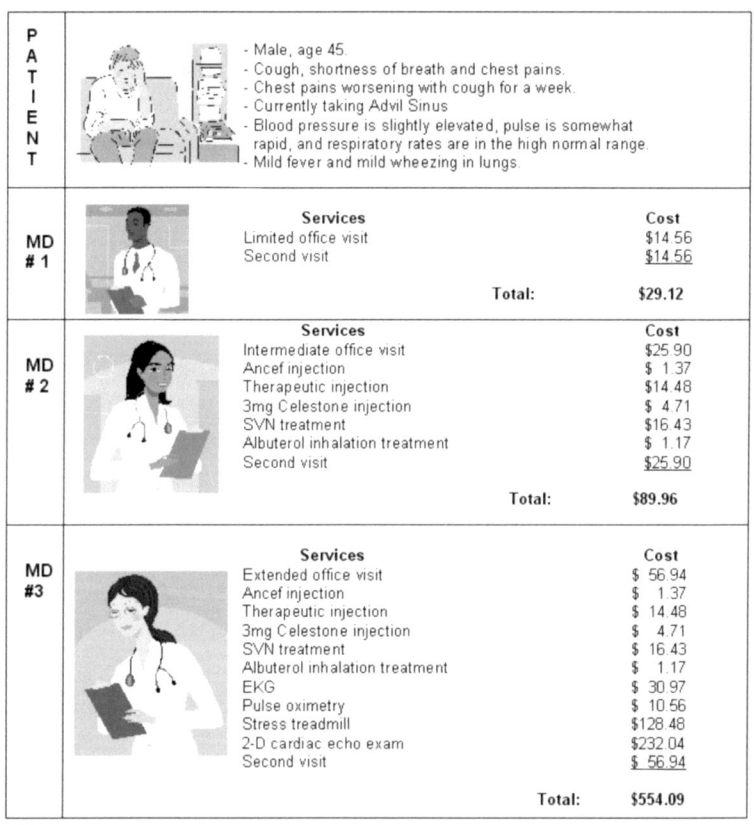

| P A T I E N T | | - Male, age 45. - Cough, shortness of breath and chest pains. - Chest pains worsening with cough for a week. - Currently taking Advil Sinus - Blood pressure is slightly elevated, pulse is somewhat rapid, and respiratory rates are in the high normal range. - Mild fever and mild wheezing in lungs. | |
|---|---|---|---|
| MD # 1 | | **Services** Limited office visit Second visit | **Cost** $14.56 $14.56 |
| | | **Total:** | **$29.12** |
| MD # 2 | | **Services** Intermediate office visit Ancef injection Therapeutic injection 3mg Celestone injection SVN treatment Albuterol inhalation treatment Second visit | **Cost** $25.90 $ 1.37 $14.48 $ 4.71 $16.43 $ 1.17 $25.90 |
| | | **Total:** | **$89.96** |
| MD #3 | | **Services** Extended office visit Ancef injection Therapeutic injection 3mg Celestone injection SVN treatment Albuterol inhalation treatment EKG Pulse oximetry Stress treadmill 2-D cardiac echo exam Second visit | **Cost** $ 56.94 $ 1.37 $ 14.48 $ 4.71 $ 16.43 $ 1.17 $ 30.97 $ 10.56 $128.48 $232.04 $ 56.94 |
| | | **Total:** | **$554.09** |

Source: Controlling Health Care Costs (Gilbertson, 2005)

The costs shown are estimates of what each service would cost the Hotel Employees and Restaurant Employees International Union Welfare Fund and do not include the costs of any medicines that the doctors recommended the patient take after and/or in between visits with the patient. Each doctor was then told that the patient would have been found to have Viral

10

Bronchitis, which would seem to suggest that along with a prescription for an antibiotic, physician number one's treatment plan would have been sufficient and resulted in a cured patient. One of the most noteworthy aspects of this case study is the increasing use of medical technology by each physician as the treatment became more complex including injections, inhalation treatments, EKGs, even a stress treadmill and a cardiac echo exam. As the treatment became more complex, the cost to the insurance company (and likely the insured considering co pays, transportation costs for the repeated visits, missed work for the procedures, etc.) increased dramatically. Physician number three's total treatment cost is over six times more expensive than that of physician number two's, who proposed a treatment plan over three times more expensive than physician number one's, which in the end along with a prescription would have been adequate (Gilbertson, 2005).

Dr. Ani Aprahamian, PhD, a Professor of Experimental Nuclear Physics at the University of Notre Dame, in her Presentation on Positron Emission Tomography (PET) identifies multiple real life cases where PET scans were able to improve the treatment of patients where diagnosis was initially done using other technology. Those improvements came in the form of preventing unnecessary procedures and decreasing costs to the patient, insurance company and all parties involved. Here is a summary of two of those cases Dr. Aprahamian described in detail:

## Case Study 1

A 71 year old male is discovered to have metastic melanoma on his left shoulder. A CT scan 6 months later reveals another tumor in his distal demur and adjacent soft tissue but no findings in his abdomen. A bone scan days later shows the femur tumor and four spine lesions. The patient is scheduled for an amputation. However, a whole-body PET scan is performed and numerous lesions are found throughout the body. Surgery is cancelled. The cost and trauma of the operation is avoided as the surgery would have been ineffective.

## Case Study 2

A 63 year old male has lung cancer. A tumor has been removed from his right lung's upper lobe. Several months later a CT scan shows a lesion on his left lung. However, a PET scan is performed and focal FDG accumulation is found in the left long but in addition several other lesions previously undetected are seen in the right lung and his mediastinal lymph nodes as well. The patient' treatment is immediately switched to chemotherapy.

In both cases, the more costly and technologically advanced PET scan did not only produce better results for diagnosis and treatment, unnecessary and/or ineffective procedures were averted. While we do not know if there was actually any cost benefit, given these patients were also subjected to other costly forms of diagnosis, we can see through these case studies that advanced medical technology when applied correctly can produce highly desirable results for patients (Aprahamian, n.d.).

## Discussion and Future Directions

As we see from the literature review and case studies presented in this paper, these is compelling evidence that advances in medical technology and medical technology itself contributes, among many other factors to rising health care costs. We've also observed some of the root causes contributing to medical technology's effect in this regard. There are many avenues that can be pursued for future directions of research. One of the most beneficial may be following up on the suggestions of Dr. Rita Redberg, M.D. of the University of California, San Francisco's Medical Center with regards to developing a system tht truly looks at the costs of new medical technologies emerging and post-emergance and in their acceptance phases, determining the benefits and ensuring they outweigh the commonly high costs associated with the new equipment, drugs, etc. According to Dr. Redberg that review and research, like in many other countries should be the responsibility of government.

Another avenue of research that may yield interesting results would be the study of how the United States compares to other nations of similar population size both with and without Universal Healthcare systems in place. Some of the literature reviewed in this paper contained comparisons to other nations, however much more could be done to provide a variety of results for comparison. However, it does appear to be incorrect to assume that under a Universal Healthcare system advances in medical technology would not contribute to any rises in health care costs. Despite which entitity is paying for these advances, specifically the high cost of new technology when introduced, government or private insurance company, the cost will still exist.

## Conclusions

In conclusion, there is a large amount of literature that has touched on the impact of medical technology and advances on the rising health care costs in the United States. There are an equal number of explanations for the impact. However there is no clear and concise plan to combat this. In fact, combating it almost seems contra productive to the advancement of medicine, the improvement of the quality of life and the increasing life span of humans. Some experts do appear to agree though that the better approach to increasing costs due to advances in medical technology is to better regulate the implementation and the use of high cost medical technology such that the benefit for the cost is maximized to provide an effective solution.

# References

Gilbertson, E. (2005). Controlling health care costs presentation to The Citizen's Health Care Working Group 2005 Conference. Salt Lake City, UT.

Aprahamian, A. (n.d.). Presentation on Positron Emission Tomography (PET). Online Directory, Medical Physics. University of Notre Dame. http://www.nd.edu/~aapraham/MedicalPhys/

NCHC, National Coalition on Health Care. (2007) *Facts on the Cost of Health Care.* Retrieved April 01, 2008 from http://www.nchc.org/facts/cost.shtml

Harvard University Survey/The USA Today/Kaiser Family Foundation Project. (August 2005). *Health Care Costs Survey.* Kaiser Family Foundation's Publication # 7371. http://www.kff.org

Barros, A. (1995). How labs contribute to rising health care costs. *Medical Laboratory Observer, February 1995 volume*, 1-4.

News-Medical.net (2007). Advancing medical technology increases health-care costs. *News-Medical.net Medical News Service. January 9, 2007 edition,* 1-2.

Lohr, S. (2004, September 26). Health care costs are a killer, but maybe that's a plus. *The New York Times,* pp. 1, 2, 3.

University Of Michigan (1998, August 19). New medical technology may override health care costs. *ScienceDaily.* Retrieved March 24, 2008, from http://www.sciencedaily.com /releases/1998/08/980819080823.htm

Bodenheimer, T. (2005). High and rising healthcare costs. *Medicine and Public Issues Journal.* Volume 142, Number 11

Olund, P. (2008, April 07). Timeline of medical breakthroughs. *Channel One Network.*
Retrieved April 16, 2008 from
http://www.channelone.com/news/2005/12/02/medicine_history

Long, T. (2007, December 24). Dec. 24, 1936: Radiation used to treat disease for the first
time. *WIRED.* Retrieved March 14, 2008 from:
http://www.wired.com/science/discoveries/news/2007/12/dayintech_1224

Cancer Research UK Charity (2007, June 14). Who discovered chemotheraphy? *Cancer
Research UK Charity.* Retrieved April 5, 2008 from:
http://www.cancerhelp.org.uk/help/default.asp?page=2598

Reggio E. (n.d.). Stages of Medicine. *Personal Website of Reggio Emilia, PhD.*
Retrieved April 09, 2008 from: http://www.vency.com/defeateddiseases.html

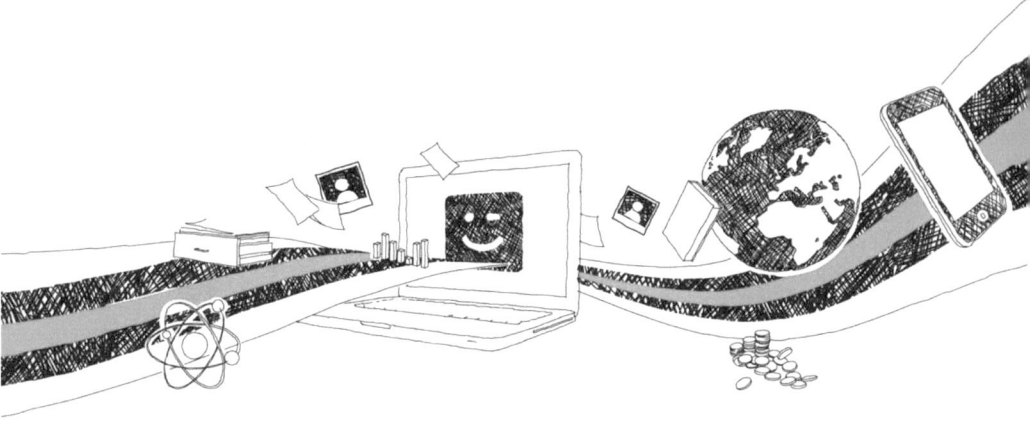
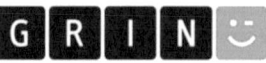